Herbal Supplements

Top 10 Herbal Supplements and Their Benefits

By: Bring On Fitness

© Copyright 2018 – Bring On Fitness – All Rights Reserved.

Table of Contents

About Bring On Fitness

Our passion for fitness gave life to **Bring On Fitness**. We started with the goal of helping as many people as we can. To educate, motivate and to help change peoples lives for the better. Bring On Fitness is not only for the fitness enthusiasts, but also for the beginner. We strongly believe nothing is more important than learning the basics and creating a strong foundation in both nutrition - through meal planning, and in exercise - by following a specific plan. This is just as important for the beginner, as it is for the experienced athlete.

We set high standards for ourselves, the information we share, and the products we carry. Our goal is to provide you with exceptional products that suit your needs and the knowledge and motivation to help you work towards and achieve your health and fitness goals.

Keep up to date by liking us on Facebook and Instagram @bringonfitness

And for a complete list of reads and a FREE GIFT check us out at: www.bringonfitness.com

"Our Mission is to have a positive impact in changing peoples lives. We will deliver the best possible fitness and nutrition solutions that will empower people to achieve their health and fitness goals."

Introduction

I want to thank you for choosing this book, *"Herbal Supplements: Top 10 Herbal Supplements and Their Benefits."*

Did you know that more than 25% of the drugs that we use these days are derived from plants? The World Health Organization has a list of 252 essential medicines, and of this, 11 % are exclusively derived from plants.

Morphine is a necessary medicine in the medical field and was discovered about 200 years ago. This powerful medicine is made from the seedpods of the poppy flower. Since then, scientists have started actively studying different plants and their properties that can be used to create various pharmaceutical products. However, after years of overmedication, people have started to understand the benefits of natural or herbal medicines.

In this book, you will learn about the top 10 herbal supplements, their benefits, and the simple ways in which you can include these ingredients in your daily diet. If you want to improve your overall health but you don't want any synthesized supplements, then this is the best book for you.

I sincerely hope you find the book informative and helpful in your quest to understand more about herbal supplements.

Thank you once again for choosing this book. Let us get started!

Chapter One: About Herbal Supplements

Millions of dollars go into the research of medicinal herbs. The use of traditional herbal supplements is still modest when compared to the use of manufactured pharmaceutical medicines. However, all the research and investment in the field of herbal medicines indicate a shift in the general outlook towards alternative and natural forms of treatment.

Human history is peppered with instances of usage of natural plant products for different reasons. In fact, the earliest written record of herbal medicine goes back to more than 5000 years ago. For our early ancestors, herbal medicine was the only form of treatment. Nowadays, a lot of plant-based compounds are regularly used to treat different health conditions, such as allergies, arthritis, skin infections, wounds, gastrointestinal issues, some forms of cancer, migraines, and so on.

Food is medicine, and the sooner we realize this, the sooner we can improve our health. Herbal medicines are cheaper and safer. Therefore, it is no wonder that a lot of people want to opt for traditional practices of medicine instead of modern ones.

So, what is herbal medicine? Herbal medicine uses plants and naturally occurring plant-based substances to treat illnesses. These products are often a mixture of different organic compounds that are present in raw or processed parts of certain plants. Herbal medicine is a part of different cultures across the world. There are various systems of herbal medicine, as well as philosophy and practices, and each of these systems is influenced by different social, environmental, and geographic conditions. The one thing that they all share is their holistic approach towards life and medicine.

If you use healing herbs, you can improve your overall health. Botanical medicine is not a new concept; it has been around for over thousands of years and is still in practice today. Traditional Chinese medicine and Ayurveda are among the two most ancient and popular forms of herbal medicines. Most traditional medicinal practices place a great emphasis on health and not the disease.

According to the World Health Organization, over 80% of the population across the globe still relies on herbal medicine as part of their primary health care. Whole herbs contain various ingredients that help treat diseases and remove symptoms of illnesses. Herbal medicine is also known as botanical medicine, and it uses seeds, berries, leaves, roots, stems, barks, or even flowers of plants for medicinal purposes. Here are a couple of benefits that herbal supplements provide:

- They are certainly more affordable when compared with conventional medicines. Modern medicines come with a hefty price tag. One reason for the increase in the popularity of herbal medicines is that they are cost-effective.

- Herbal remedies are also more natural to obtain than any other prescription medicines. For instance, herbal extracts, such as essential oils and herbal teas, are readily available in most health food stores and even local grocery stores. You don't need a doctor's prescription to obtain these ingredients. Isn't it better to brew a cup of herbal tea to deal with a headache rather than popping a pill? All the pills and medicines we consume are helpful, but they have certain side effects as well.

- Herbs are used to treat chronic ailments and various acute medical conditions, such as cardiovascular diseases, prostate problems, depression, inflammation, and so on. Herbal medicines also help improve the overall immunity of a person.

Depression and anxiety-related disorders seem to be quite common these days. Most of us live in a constant state of stress and anxiety, thanks to our hectic lives. Chronic stress can even damage your physical and mental wellbeing. However, it is impossible to avoid stress. So what's the solution to this problem? How can you cope with anxiety and not let all things bog you down? You must realize that you have more power over stress than you believe. The right herbs can help to calm you down and reduce your stress.

Herbal medicines are beneficial. However, you must always consult your physician or doctor before you decide to try any of the herbal supplements discussed in this book.

In the next section, you will learn about the top 10 herbal supplements and their benefits. Not just that, but you will also learn about easy ways through which you can incorporate them into your daily diet to improve your overall health.

Garlic

Garlic is one of the most popular condiments that we regularly use in cooking. Did you know that garlic is a vital herb that is often used in medicinal remedies? Garlic contains different nutrients, flavonoids, selenium, allicin, sulfur, and oligosaccharides. If you like the taste and flavor of garlic, then you are in for a treat. Garlic not only adds flavor to your food, but it can also improve your overall health if you consume it raw.

Benefits

There are various health benefits that garlic offers, and they are as follows:

- It acts as a blood purifier. If you add a little garlic to your food daily, you can get rid of all those zits that bother you.

- Garlic cleanses your system of all toxins.

- Garlic also helps you to battle cold and flu. You can sip some garlic tea or eat two to three cloves of raw garlic daily.

- Garlic is rich in antioxidants, which help to reduce the levels of cholesterol in your body.

- Garlic consists of allicin; this compound regulates the levels of blood sugar and blood pressure.

- Garlic has antibacterial properties, and it treats bacterial, fungal, and parasitic infections.

- Daily consumption of garlic also prevents different forms of stomach and colorectal cancers.

- Use garlic-infused oil if you want your hair to look lustrous; however, make sure you thoroughly rinse your hair afterward!

Usage

If you want to lose weight, then add two cloves of garlic to a glass of warm water along with the juice of half a lemon. If you don't like the flavor of raw garlic, adding a couple of cloves of garlic to your food might be helpful. However, it is better to consume raw garlic if you want to reap all the benefits it offers. When you cook garlic, it tends to lose some of its medicinal properties.

Ginger

Ginger is a superfood, and it is a flowering plant. It is a common ingredient in traditional methods like Ayurveda and Chinese medicine. Ginger is one of the most popular condiments across the world. Ginger contains gingerol, and the therapeutic benefits it offers is due to this compound. Gingerol is the oily resin present in this miracle root, which works as an excellent antioxidant and has anti-inflammatory properties as well.

Benefits

- Ginger helps with digestions, relieves nausea, and fights flu and cold.

- Ginger is a popular remedy for seasickness.

- If you suffer from morning sickness, then a small cup of ginger tea can fix that problem quickly. Ginger can help treat morning sickness, nausea caused by chemotherapy, or even regular nausea.

- The next time you feel like your body is sore after exercising, use some ginger-infused oil to massage the troubled area.

- Inflammation is a severe problem that can cause a host of painful conditions like arthritis. If you want to control and treat inflammation, then you must consume a little ginger daily.

- This superfood has anti-diabetic properties. Ginger can also help reduce the risk of high blood pressure and cholesterol. It is a superfood with multiple benefits.

- Chronic indigestion causes frequent pain and discomfort in your abdominal region. Indigestion can lead to other troubles as well. You can keep all this at bay with the help of ginger.

- Ginger can also help to reduce menstrual cramps. Have a cup of ginger-infused tea to regulate your bowel movement and deal with other bodily pains.

Usage

Ginger is a common ingredient in Asian cuisine. Now that you are aware of the different benefits ginger provides, you simply need to add a little ginger to your daily diet. Ginger is a wonder root, and you can use it in different ways. You can have raw ginger, add it to tea, or even take it in powdered form. If you want to use it topically, you can use oil infused with ginger. The best way to consume ginger is to simply add a few slivers to a cup of tea. Add some lemon juice, honey, and slivers of ginger to brew a relaxing tea. If you have a sweet tooth, then you can try some candied ginger as well. The next time you decide to make some caramel, add in some finely chopped ginger. However, make sure that you don't cook the ginger. Raw ginger offers more benefits than cooked ginger. You can use raw, dried, or powdered ginger. So make sure that you stock your pantry with some ginger.

Turmeric

Turmeric has a long history of medicinal usage that dates back to over 4000 years. Only recently did modern medicine realize the importance of this wonderful plant. You can add turmeric to your food or even take it in the form of a supplement.

Benefits

There are different benefits that turmeric offers, and they are as follows:

- Turmeric has several bioactive compounds with excellent medicinal properties. Turmeric contains specific compounds known as curcuminoids. An essential curcuminoid is curcumin, and it is an active ingredient in turmeric. It is a natural antioxidant with anti-inflammatory properties. However, the body doesn't absorb curcumin easily into the bloodstream. To improve the absorption of curcumin, it is advisable to consume some pepper along with it. So swallow a couple of peppercorns along with turmeric.

- Inflammation helps your body fight off any foreign bodies in your system. Inflammation is your body's defense mechanism, and it is essential. However, too much inflammation causes a lot of problems. Long-term inflammation is not only painful, but it is quite problematic as well. Chronic inflammation can cause a host of degenerative diseases, such as cardiovascular diseases, Alzheimer's, cancer, and metabolic syndrome.

- Curcumin blocks the NF-kB molecule that triggers the genes related to inflammation in the nuclei of cells. Oxidative stress causes premature aging and other diseases. The free radicals in the body react with unpaired electrons, and this creates highly reactive molecules. These free radicals interact and react with organic substances like proteins, fatty acids, and DNA. All these cause oxidative stress. Antioxidants present in turmeric protect the body from free radicals and neutralize any oxidative stress. The curcumin present in turmeric also stimulates the production of antioxidants in your body.

- The primary cause of most brain disorders is the decrease in the levels of Brain-Derived Neurotrophic Factor (BDNF), a growth hormone. A reduction in this hormone can cause mental diseases like depression and Alzheimer's. Curcumin increases the levels of BDNF, and this improves brain health. An increase in the levels of BDNF can also improve your memory.

- The antioxidant properties of curcumin help to reverse several risk factors of cardiovascular diseases. It controls the levels of cholesterol and blood sugar. If you can manage these two factors, then you can significantly reduce the risk of cardiovascular diseases and improve heart health.

Usage

Ever wonder why certain curries have a yellow tinge? Well, turmeric is the condiment that lends a yellow color to food. It is commonly used in Asian kitchens. It is not only a spice, but it is a medicinal herb as well. You can consume turmeric in raw or powdered form. The powdered form of turmeric is quite popular and is often found in all Asian households. It is a good idea to add turmeric to a fatty meal because curcumin is fat-soluble. Turmeric is also used in topical body products. Some freshly ground turmeric can cleanse your skin, especially if you suffer from acne.

Ginseng

An extremely popular herbal medicine is ginseng. Asians and North Americans have been using this herb for centuries. Native Americans used the ginseng root to cure headaches and as treatment for infertility. The ideal consumption of ginseng is about 200 mg to 400 mg a day, depending on the ailment you want to treat.

Benefits

- Ginseng is an antioxidant, and it has anti-inflammatory properties. Ginseng extract can help reduce inflammation and improve the circulation of blood in the body. Ginseng is a household remedy for headaches. It can also help to improve the function of the brain and have a positive influence on your mood.

- If you have trouble sleeping at night, then a glass of warm milk steeped with ginseng will do the trick.

- Ginseng contains gametocides and compound K that help to repair any damage that free radicals cause. Reversals in the harmful effect of free radicals improve the brain's health.

- If you feel stressed or distracted, a cup of ginseng tea can help improve your focus and calm your mind.

- Erectile dysfunction is not an easy problem to treat, but ginseng is a great alternative to pharmaceutical drugs. Oxidative stress in the tissues and blood vessels present in the penis cause erectile dysfunction. Ginseng reverses the process of oxidative stress. Not just that, it also helps improve the circulation of blood in the penis. Therefore, it can help improve erectile dysfunction. To treat erectile dysfunction, a person might need to consume about 1000 mg of ginseng daily for at least six weeks.

- Ginseng also strengthens the immune system. It comes in handy for those dealing with degenerative diseases like cancer.

- Ginseng alleviates fatigue and improves your energy levels.

Usage

There are different ways in which you can consume ginseng. You can use dried ginseng, powdered form, or even in tablets and capsules. It is up to you and your convenience. You can brew tea with ginseng and sip it whenever you feel tired. To brew ginseng tea, add some dried ginseng to warm water, and let it simmer for a couple of minutes. You can also add it to a glass of warm milk. You can even consume raw ginseng or steam it a little.

If you like stir fries, use some ginseng to add flavor to your meal. You can add ginseng to soups and broths as well. The amount of ginseng you consume will depend on the condition you want to improve. For instance, the suggested dose of ginseng is about 1 to 2 grams per day.

Milk Thistle

The extracts of milk thistle have been used as an herbal remedy for more than 2000 years. The seeds of milk thistle contain lipophilic extracts that act as bioflavonoids. Bioflavonoids help to improve the immunity and reduce oxidative stress in the body.

Benefits

- Milk thistle is typically used to treat liver problems. Silymarin is an active ingredient present in milk thistle, and it reduces the production of free radicals. Silymarin is an antioxidant, and it reduces any damage that is caused by oxidative stress on the liver.

- It has anti-aging properties that improve the health of your skin. Aside from its anti-aging properties, it also helps with inflammatory skin conditions.

- High levels of cholesterol can wreak havoc on your cardiac health, and milk thistle reduces the level of harmful cholesterol in the body.

- Silymarin also assists in weight loss.

- If you suffer from type 2 diabetes, then milk thistle can help reduce insulin resistance in the body. If insulin resistance decreases, management of diabetes becomes easy.

- Like mentioned earlier, silymarin has anti-inflammatory properties, and it clears the airways in the body. Milk thistle can help reduce the symptoms of asthma in human beings.

- In women, the weakening of bones is a common condition caused by the lack of estrogen. Milk thistle improves bone health.

- Oxidative stress causes degenerative cellular diseases like Alzheimer's, and it improves the brain's cognitive function.

Most of the data on milk thistle comes from studies conducted on mice. However, scientists and researchers are quite confident that it will have the same effect on human health. They are not mistaken to think so. Milk thistle is used in ancient Chinese medicine and Ayurvedic medicine.

Usage

Milk thistle extracts are easily available in the form of capsules, and you can take these capsules as supplements. You can use oil infused with milk thistle topically to improve the health of your skin. Milk thistle can help improve your overall health and immunity. You can always consume milk thistle in the form of tea as well, or you can add a couple of drops of milk thistle extract to your regular cup of tea. If you want to use this medicinal herb, then take one teaspoon of milk thistle seeds, and grind them in a coffee grinder. Steep the ground seeds in 175 ml or 6 fl oz of boiling water for about five to 10 minutes. Alternatively, if you can obtain fresh stalks of milk thistle, you can soak them overnight in water and then boil them until tender. These can be consumed with a little butter and salt.

Feverfew

If you suffer from chronic migraines and headaches, then feverfew is a safe alternative to pharmaceutical drugs. If you want a natural remedy to treat migraines, then read on. The best thing about this herb is that you can easily grow it in your kitchen garden. You no longer need to search for fresh feverfew if you want to brew a headache-relieving concoction.

Benefits

- The most common use of feverfew is to deal with migraines and headaches.

- It is a natural painkiller and has certain anti-inflammatory properties. It contains a compound that reduces the secretion of serotonin, an inflammatory agent in the blood vessels. It also slows down the secretion of histamine, a chemical transmitter.

- A pulsating headache and nausea are the common symptoms of the onset of a migraine, and feverfew reduces these symptoms quite effectively.

- Feverfew also reduces the damage caused to skin by eczema and dermatitis. If you want younger and better-looking skin, then you must certainly try feverfew.

- Feverfew impairs the production of prostaglandin and reverses the action of neutrophils in the body. A combination of these two actions helps it to reduce any inflammation in the body that an autoimmune disease usually causes.

- Menstrual cramps are quite common, and most of the women experience them. Whenever the lining of the uterus produces an excess of prostaglandin, it causes pain and inflammation. Given that feverfew reduces the production of prostaglandin in the body, it indirectly reduces the pain that menstrual cramps cause.

- It also reduces blood pressure. Feverfew reduces pain because it helps reduce inflammation in the body.

Usage

You can find feverfew supplements in the form of capsules, tablets, and liquid extracts. The supplements are either made of fresh or dried feverfew. The parthenolide content is used to measure the standard dosage of feverfew, and the advised dosage must contain about 0.2 parthenolide. To reduce a migraine in an adult, you need to take 100 mg to 300 mg of feverfew at least three times daily. You can use the leaves of feverfew to brew tea as well. However, these leaves are quite bitter and can leave an odd aftertaste in your mouth. So you can sweeten them up with a little honey.

St. John's Wort

This herb is a popular antidepressant, and humans have been using it in traditional medicine for over 2000 years. It produces biologically active substances like hypericin and hyperforin. These two compounds alleviate the symptoms of various health conditions.

Benefits

- Perhaps the most popular benefit of this herb is in the treatment of depression. It is a natural antidepressant, and it relieves the symptoms of depression. You no longer need to visit a doctor or take medication to handle depression. A mild brew of St. John's Wort will instantly uplift your mood. However, it is used only to treat mild and moderate cases and not instances of chronic depression.

- St. John's Wort inhibits the secretion of harmful neurotransmitters like dopamine, serotonin, and norepinephrine that cause depression. It not only helps with depression, but it also reduces mood swings and anxiety.

- It regulates the hormonal balance in the body and regularizes your sleep cycle. A cup of tea steeped with St. John's Wort can immediately reduce any fatigue you experience.

- Addiction to nicotine, tobacco, and alcohol are difficult to overcome. This herb eases the withdrawal symptoms that a person might face while trying to overcome an addiction.

Usage

To treat moderate to low levels of depression, the ideal dosage is about 300 mg of St. John's Wort thrice a day. The standard hypericin content in St. John's Wort extract needs to be about 0.2% to 0.3%. This herb is also used to treat the symptoms of menopause. You need to take about 0.2 mg/ml hypericin to reduce the symptoms of menopause. You can consume teas brewed with St. John's Wort to treat any of the ailments that it cures. Alternatively, it is also available in the form of liquid extracts that you can add to water and consume. It is often used in salves and balms to reduce any skin irritation. Topical creams with St. John's Wort will improve the health of your skin. You can brew a tea using this herb, just like chamomile. Whenever you want to make a savory broth or a stock, you can use water infused with St. John's wort.

Ginkgo Biloba

Ginkgo biloba is commonly known as maidenhair, and it is frequently used in traditional Chinese medicine. The scientific name of ginkgo biloba is salisburia adiantifolia. It is the extract from the Chinese ginkgo tree. Several studies about the vitality of this herb are being conducted. Dried ginkgo leaves, as well as seeds, are used in herbal remedies. Ginkgo biloba contains two important compounds, and these are flavonoids and terpenoids. These two compounds are responsible for all the benefits that this herb provides.

Benefits

- Ginkgo biloba is a natural antidepressant, and it helps control mild forms of depression and alleviates mood swings.

- It balances the hormonal levels in your body.

- The extracts of ginkgo biloba improve the cognitive functions of the brain. A cup of tea with ginkgo biloba extracts can enhance your focus and level of concentration.

- Ginkgo biloba extracts also help treat several mental and cognitive disorders like Alzheimer's and dementia. It reverses the effect of neurodegenerative diseases and improves the brain's health.

- Ginkgo biloba also enhances blood circulation and slows down the process of aging.

Usage

To treat any problems related to memory degeneration, you need to consume about 120 mg to 240 mg of this herb daily. The dosage needs to contain about 25% of flavonoids and 10% of terpenoids. The same dosage can also reduce fatigue and mood swings. It will take about five to six weeks to see a positive change in your overall wellbeing. Make sure that you consume the ginkgo biloba extract daily. However, if you suffer from chronic depression or any other serious disease, you must consult your doctor before you use this herbal remedy. Ginkgo biloba extracts are also available in the form of capsules and tablets that you can take as supplements.

Saw Palmetto

The scientific name of this herb is Serenoa repens. Only the dark purple berries of this plant are used in medicinal treatments. Saw palmetto could grow as either a tree or a lush shrub with green leaves. It is native to the West Indies and the United States. The active ingredients present in Saw Ppalmetto include fatty acids, sterols, and flavonoids.

Benefits

- Saw palmetto improves the texture and health of the hair.

- It is used in treatments for impotence. It enhances the libido and promotes the overall sexual health of a person.

- It also helps treat kidney disorders and lowers the risk of cancer.

- It increases muscle mass. If you want to improve your overall immunity, then this is an excellent herb to try.

Usage

You can buy dried saw palmetto berries at any health store. Saw palmetto is also available in the form of capsules, tablets, and tinctures. The simplest way to consume this herb is to steep it into a cup of tea. The recommended dosage of saw palmetto depends on the condition you want to treat. For instance, if you're going to use this herb to treat Benign Prostatic Hypertrophy (BPH), then you need to consume about three doses of 320 mg of saw palmetto daily. The most effective way to consume saw palmetto is in capsule form. You can brew a pot of tea with it, but you need to understand that the active ingredient in it is a fatty acid, and it isn't soluble in water. Saw palmetto is not safe for consumption for pregnant and breastfeeding women. Always consult your doctor before you decide to use this remedy.

Aloe Vera

Aloe vera contains different vitamins and minerals that improve your overall health and body functions. It contains vitamins A, C, E, and B12. Apart from these, aloe vera also contains folic acid and choline. There are eight active enzymes present in it: aliiase, alkaline phosphate, amylase, cellulase, lipase, peroxidase, carboxypeptidase, and bradykinesia. Apart from all this, it contains minerals, natural laxatives, fatty acids, and helpful sugars. It is quite easy to find products with aloe in them. However, if you want to reap the benefits that this miracle herb provides, then it is better to use fresh aloe vera.

Benefits

- Aloe is typically used to treat rashes and skin irritations. In fact, it is the best cure for sunburn. Aside from treating sunburn, you can also use aloe gel to treat any burn injuries you sustain.

- It helps heal cold sores because aloe is safe for oral consumption. The moisturizing properties of aloe improve the health of the skin and hair.

- It also improves digestion and treats constipation.

Usage

It is quite easy to grow aloe vera, and you can grow it in your kitchen garden. The succulent leaves of aloe contain all the magical ingredients that improve a person's health. Aloe is safe to consume, and you can add it to your smoothies. However, make sure that you don't expose aloe to any heat. Heat destroys the fatty acids and hormones present in it. You can add aloe juice to your shampoo and toothpaste. Aloe can also be added to moisturizers to improve your skin's health. If you have irritable skin or want to treat any inflammatory skin conditions, rub some fresh aloe gel on the affected area.

Natural remedies that contain herbs are much better than the pharmaceuticals we consume today. Herbal medicine dates back to more than 5000 years. In fact, herbalism is steadily gaining popularity these days. It is cost-effective, has several health benefits, and has no side effects. However, make sure that you consult your healthcare provider before you decide to use any of the herbal remedies provided in this book.

Conclusion

I want to thank you once again for purchasing this book.

Herbal medicine has plenty of benefits, but the most important one is that the lack of synthetic compounds doesn't harm your health. Natural remedies are cheap, readily available, and don't have the side effects of modern drugs. You need to understand the benefits of different herbal supplements and the ways to use them. Once you have sufficient knowledge of these two things, the next step is to use them regularly.

All the information provided in this book will help you with this. Now that you know the different natural supplements that can improve your health and treat ailments naturally, all that you need to do is include these miracle ingredients in your diet.

Thank you, and remember to share how well these xxx tips work for you. You can do that by writing a review in your Amazon account under Your Orders.

Thank you,

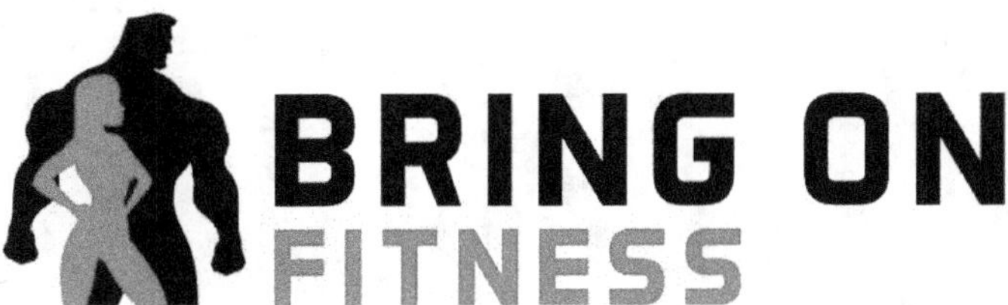

Sources

https://draxe.com/herbal-medicine/

https://food.ndtv.com/food-drinks/powerhouse-of-medicine-and-flavour-surprising-health-benefits-of-garlic-1200468

https://www.healthline.com/nutrition/11-proven-benefits-of-ginger#section11

https://www.healthline.com/nutrition/top-10-evidence-based-health-benefits-of-turmeric#section10

https://www.healthline.com/nutrition/ginseng-benefits#section1

https://www.medicalnewstoday.com/articles/320362.php

https://www.thealternativedaily.com/benefits-of-feverfew/

https://www.organicfacts.net/health-benefits/herbs-and-spices/st-johns-wort.html

About Bring On Fitness

Our passion for fitness gave life to **Bring On Fitness**. We started with the goal of helping as many people as we can. To educate, motivate and to help change peoples lives for the better. Bring On Fitness is not only for the fitness enthusiasts, but also for the beginner. We strongly believe nothing is more important than learning the basics and creating a strong foundation in both nutrition - through meal planning, and in exercise - by following a specific plan. This is just as important for the beginner, as it is for the experienced athlete.

We set high standards for ourselves, the information we share, and the products we carry. Our goal is to provide you with exceptional products that suit your needs and the knowledge and motivation to help you work towards and achieve your health and fitness goals.

Keep up to date by liking us on Facebook and Instagram @bringonfitness

And for a complete list of reads and a FREE GIFT check us out at: www.bringonfitness.com

"Our Mission is to have a positive impact in changing peoples lives. We will deliver the best possible fitness and nutrition solutions that will empower people to achieve their health and fitness goals."